JASMINE LARUE

I WIN!

THE JOURNEY OF RECEIVING HEALING AND WALKING IN VICTORY

I WIN
The Journey of Receiving Healing and Walking in Victory

JASMINE LaRUE
jnlarue24@gmail.com

ISBN 978-1-943342-32-7

Printed in the USA.
All rights reserved

Published by: Destined To Publish | Flossmoor, Illinois
www.DestinedToPublish.com

Dedication

I would first like to dedicate this book to my Lord and Savior Jesus Christ. Without Him, I wouldn't be here. God has been better to me than I could ever be to myself. He has healed me, comforted me, and provided for me. God is my everything! Thank you, God, for opening doors for me. I am forever grateful.

Next, I dedicate this book to my younger sister Zykia, who, without hesitation, donated her kidney to me! I admire the way you love others and how hardworking you are. Thank you for being a listening ear, loving me, being supportive, and overall giving me great advice. Thank you for being level-headed and an inspiration to me. I appreciate you, and I love you very much.

Finally, I would like to dedicate this book to my parents. They have given me a tremendous support system throughout my entire life. They have been there for me physically, financially, spiritually, and emotionally. Thank you for all of your love and support. I appreciate you both so much. I love you so much.

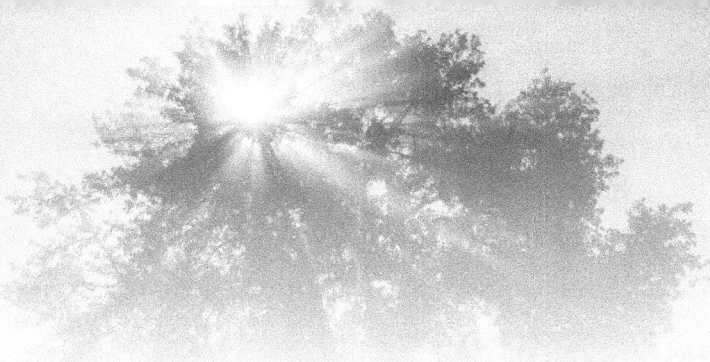

Acknowledgments

I would first like to acknowledge my older sister Tyesha. Thank you, Tyesha, for being with me the times I was in the hospital. Thank you for praying for me. All your efforts reminded me of what God says about me. Thank you for interceding for me, being supportive, and overall, being a great sister.

I want to say thank you to my little brother Anthony for always being there and doing more than what was expected of him. Thank you for the love you have for me.

I would like to thank my friend Chaunte and her children for helping me immensely, from driving my car to helping me clean and pack my apartment. You and the kids are amazing, and I truly appreciate you all.

Another big thanks goes to Apostle Regina Stevenson for staying with me while I was in the hospital. Thank you for your prayers, for interceding for me, and for always being there for me. Thank you for your teaching and reminding me what God's Word says so that I can speak the Word of God for myself in difficult situations. I am truly grateful and appreciate you very much.

Last, but certainly not least, I would like to acknowledge my friends and family for their prayers, gifts, and words of encouragement. Thank you.

Contents

Introduction

What is the definition of "win"? According to Webster's dictionary, "to win" "means to be successful or victorious in a contest or conflict ". Many times in our lives, we find ourselves struggling with or through different situations and trials, whether it's physically, financially, mentally, spiritually, or even in our relationships. One thing is for sure: if God has given you the victory in one situation or area of your life, then He will be faithful and just to give you victory in ANY situation you find yourself in. Isaiah 53:5 (New International Version) says, *"But he was pierced for our transgressions, he was crushed for our iniquities; the punishment that brought us peace was on him, and by his wounds we are healed."* We have to know and believe that every stripe that Jesus received was for every sickness, disease, pain, and hurt that we could ever experience. There is no physical pain or sickness or emotional wound or pain that God is not prepared or equipped to heal you from.

Matthew 4:23 (NIV) states that *"Jesus went through Galilee, teaching in their synagogues, proclaiming the good news of the Kingdom, and healing every disease and sickness among the people."* Let's highlight the word EVERY in the verse. Merriam-Webster defines the word "every" as "being each individual or part of a group." Therefore, the verse says that Jesus healed every disease and sickness, meaning he healed them WITHOUT EXCEPTION! This still applies to us today, because the same God who was healing back then is still in the healing business today, and no infirmity is too difficult for God to heal. I am certainly a testimony of this.

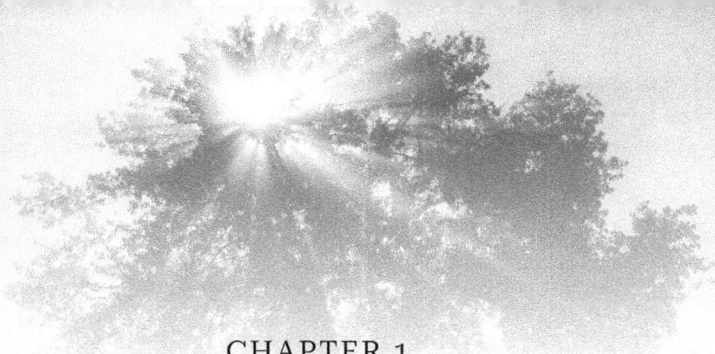

CHAPTER 1

My Health Journey

I had always believed that, when it came to my physical ability, I was treated like a typical child and adolescent. I did what most children did. I participated in sports activities and all the normal things that children do. I have always been short in stature. The only time I can even remotely remember being the same height as my peers was in kindergarten. It was something that never really bothered me until high school.

The summer before my junior year in high school, I had to get a sports physical for band and softball, so as usual my mom took me and my sister to our appointment. The doctor kept saying he didn't understand why my height and weight were so off, why I was extremely short for my age and too heavy for my height. I was always self-conscious about my weight, but I just ignored my feelings. During the appointment, my doctor told me and my mom that he was referring me to an endocrinologist and geneticist.

I started to feel a little nervous because I had no idea what that meant or what those doctors even did, but I was ready to find out what was going on. So we went to see the endocrinologist and the geneticist. I remember they were trying to get bloodwork and they had such a hard time getting a vein that they had to go through a vein in my ankle. That was one of the worst experiences I've ever had with a blood draw, and after that it was extremely hard for any other doctor or nurse to get blood from me because it was very traumatic. After all the poking and prodding, the test results came back, and the doctor informed us that I had Turner syndrome. My parents and I were shocked, confused, and concerned all at the same time, because none of us had never heard of this syndrome before and didn't know what this meant.

Here is a quick biology lesson: males are born with one X and one Y chromosome; females are born with two X chromosomes. Turner syndrome is a chromosomal disorder in which a female is born with one X chromosome instead of two. I was born with one X chromosome. According to the doctor, I was supposed to have all kinds of deficits and issues, so all the doctors who saw me were shocked because the only issue they saw was my short stature. I give all glory and honor to God because according to doctors I'm supposed to have webbed feet, and intellectual and cognitive issues, but I do not.

One treatment the doctors suggested to me and my parents was growth hormones. I also had not had my menstrual cycle come during this time, so another issue they wanted to check was my menses and my reproductive system. They informed me that women with Turner syndrome don't have the number of eggs that normal women have and that I therefore most likely wouldn't be able to have children of my own. This news was very disheartening because I've always wanted to have my own kids. I love kids and always have. Ever since I was old enough to babysit, I have helped others take care of their kids, so this news really made me sad. They did, however, put me on birth control, which induced my menstrual cycle, but after a while I noticed I was getting some blood clots with my menstruation, so I stopped taking the birth control medication.

My parents and I decided not to get the growth hormone treatments. I continued going to school and graduated high school and went on to college and was thriving. The medical professionals couldn't believe I was doing as well as I was. This was proof that God had/has a great purpose for my life. God is so amazing because even though I was diagnosed with Turner syndrome, I didn't look like or have the symptoms of a typical Turner syndrome patient. The endocrinologist then asked me if I ever did public speaking. I told her I was on a speech team, and she stated that I should think about talking to other girls with the same issue. I thank God for giving me the victory because eventhough the doctors had given me a diagnosis I didn't have the " typical symptoms". Honestly, that was the first time I had really talked in depth about my Turner syndrome diagnosis. I would get questions about why I was short, and I would tell people I have Turner syndrome, and when I went to a doctor or a physician I hadn't seen before, I would have to tell them about it. Outside my family, I had told only a couple of people up to this point. I went through high school, graduated, went to college, and lived a normal life. I graduated from college in 2012.

Little did I know my next battle would come in 2013. I had just graduated from college in the spring of 2012 with a bachelor's degree in biology. My older sister, who was living in North Carolina, informed me that the sciences were really growing and booming around the Raleigh / Durham area. So in 2013 I moved to North Carolina. I wanted to get a job in a laboratory, but because I didn't have any field or internship experience, it was hard and became stressful trying to find a job in my field. I cried almost every day. I honestly wanted to go back home to Pennsylvania, but at the same time, I didn't want to give up.

One night I started having a hard time breathing. I tossed and turned for a while and went back and forth to the bathroom. I finally went to my sister's room, and she asked me if I needed to go to the hospital. I remember nodding yes. She took me to the hospital, where I learned that my blood pressure was extremely high and my oxygen low. The doctors then informed me that I was experiencing congestive heart failure. I really didn't know what that meant. I was very scared, especially since my parents were in a different state. I am so glad that I had my older sister and brother there to help me.

I was in the hospital for a little over a week. The doctors prescribed me a cocktail of blood pressure medicine. After I was discharged, I was prescribed some blood pressure medicine, and I started to recover. Exodus 23:25 (NIV) states, "*Worship the Lord your God, and his blessing will be on your food and water. I will take away sickness from among you.*" God did just tha ! During this time I wasn't actively participating in a church. This situation really caused me to realize how good God had been to me and how His hand of protection had continued to be on me.

I then joined the church my sister was attending, and Sunday services and Bible study reignited my relationship with God. I say "reignited" because I grew up knowing about God and going to church. The difference was I was learning about and building an intimate relationship with the Father on my own. I never wanted to miss a Sunday service or Bible study. I would get very upset and cry if I had to miss. Eventually I came to the realization that having to miss church occasionally was okay and that God still loved me. I started to become more active in the church. I was teaching Children's Church on Sundays. I also started ministering in dance not only within my church but also in the community with a local community dance ministry.

Also, during this time I was working for a local convenience store, and I was constantly on my feet. I started to have some pain in my feet to the point that I could barely walk from my car to my front door. Sometimes, if they were home, I would call and ask my sister, brother, or nieces to help me. Most times because of my schedule, I would slowly shuffle my way into the house by the grace of God! One night I had arrived home from work, and my feet were hurting so, and I couldn't call anyone to come and help me. I just remember saying something like "Lord, you're going to have to help me because I can't do this by myself." So I got out of my car and started walking up our driveway, which was on an incline. As I began to walk, I felt someone holding me up, and I made it to the steps and inside the door. I knew and still know that was NOBODY BUT THE LORD who helped me that night!

The next morning, I couldn't wait to tell my sister what I had experienced. That experience was so amazing, and it really solidified the fact that God was covering me and is always with me. After a lot of prayer and a visit to a podiatrist, the pain in my feet went away, glory to God! This also reminded me that no matter how small or big the battle is, the VICTORY belongs to the Lord and that, because He gets the victory and I belong to Him, I also receive the victory. Fast forward to a few months later while at work. I was at the cash register, and I remember not feeling that great and feeling a little lightheaded, but I continued to push through and work. The next thing I remember is lying on the ground and hearing my boss and coworkers calling my name. My boss then called the ambulance and my sister. I went to the emergency room, and they had to get blood, but they were having a hard time, so they had to go through my groin to get the blood. They ran other tests and determined that I had had a syncope episode. Through it all God kept me; I didn't hit my head, and I wasn't severely injured. That was another battle and another victory because of God's faithfulness and love for me.

CHAPTER 2

Being Refined in The Fire

God had certainly healed me, and I was doing well and was serving at church, ministering in dance. I had started transitioning from working at the convenience store and was working at a great preschool. Not everything was perfect; I had some financial issues arise here and there, such as keeping and affording health insurance, but even then, God still provided and protected me. I moved into my own place. I was working two jobs because I had not quit the convience store. The Lord continued to bless me. A year later I moved into a nicer place, and I then started to pray and ask God what He wanted me to do. After a while God put in my heart to branch out and start my own childcare business. I wasn't quite sure exactly the right time to leave, but God knew. Things started to become very uncomfortable at work, and others were leaving. When I told coworkers that I was planning to leave, some told me, "You aren't going anywhere," as if they didn't believe I would actually leave.

Things at work became particularly uncomfortable, and I remember hearing the Lord tell me to put in my two weeks' notice. I was so hesitant and a little scared, but that Monday I gave the owner of the preschool my two-week notice. I didn't know what was next, but I trusted that God had me. About a week or so after my last day of work, I started watching some children on my own. It went well, my clients were awesome, and then, after a while, I started to nanny.

In late summer of 2019, I got sick. It was like a typical cold: I had some congestion and coughing. I seemed to get over it. I started to notice I was getting tired a lot faster, especially when it came to ministering in dance. I would dance to half a song and be completely wiped out, but I kept dancing. I kept going to rehearsals, and I was also still nannying. The house where I nannied had steep stairs, and I started noticing that it was a little more work to climb their stairs than normal. As time went on, I thought I was getting better but then...

In the fall it got bad. I wasn't quite sure what was going on with me. I just knew something wasn't right. I lived in a second-floor apartment. I found that I couldn't walk up the stairs without feeling like I was going to pass out or actually passing out. It had gotten to the point where I couldn't walk long distances without getting sick. Even walking up the stairs at my sister's house became hard. I remember praying when I would drive up to my apartment that I would have enough energy to make it up the stairs. It was like I used all the energy I had just to get up there. There were several times where I would make it up to my apartment, open my door, and just fall to the floor.

Driving became difficult as well. I would have to open my door at a stop sign or a traffic light so that I could vomit. I had a friend I'd run errands with, and many times I would pick her up and tell her she had to drive. My friend would call me and see if I needed anything. She is the only person who had any idea about how bad I was feeling. If she was with me, she would help carry my groceries upstairs to my apartment. I was also coughing a lot. I thought I had bronchitis. Then my legs began to swell, and I barely could walk up to my apartment. I finally told my sister to take me to the ER. We ended up going to urgent care, and they did an EKG. When the nurse came in with my vitals and EKG, he said my blood pressure was extremely high, my EKG was abnormal, and I immediately needed to go to the hospital.

I was scared. The people at the urgent care told me and my sister that I could ride to the hospital in the ambulance or have my sister transport me. I had my sister take me, and during this time I was able to pray and have others pray for me. We arrived at the hospital, and of course, my sister was there but my Apostle came as well. I had gotten to the hospital, but they didn't have a room to put me in. I was put on a bed in the hallway, and they started to draw blood and run tests while I was waiting for a room. I was eventually put into a room, where they ran more tests. I was in the hospital for a week. They couldn't explain why my blood pressure was 200+ over 100. The doctor ended up giving me three blood pressure medicines. I started to feel better, and I was discharged. A couple of weeks went by, and I was still coughing a little, and I started having some reactions, so they switched up and adjusted some of my medications.

The medications had started working, and I was recovering. The Almighty DID IT AGAIN! This takes us to the previous scripture, Exodus 23:25. I continued to dance before the Lord, and after getting out of the hospital, whether it was rehearsing, ministering in dance, or just worshiping in my home, every time I would feel sick, pass out, or be unable to stand, I would hear God in a clear voice say, "Dance," or He would say, "Just worship," and I would. Therefore, no matter the situation or circumstance, always remember that worship is your weapon against the enemy and to always follow the leading/prompting of the Holy Spirit.

I continued with my healing process even though I wasn't 100 percent. I was still having a hard time climbing stairs. My legs were still swelling. I heard the Lord tell me to go back home (Pennsylvania). I didn't understand it. God knew I really didn't want to go back home, but I said, "Okay, Lord" (at the same time asking, "Lord, are You sure?"). Months went by, and it just seemed like everything was going crazy--my finances, my business, and my health. I was going back and forth to the doctors and the cardiologist. The cardiologist ran some tests and told me he thought that I had a hole in my heart and that he didn't understand why my blood pressure was still high. He also said I might have to have heart surgery to fix it. I remember calling my mom right away and crying, and my mother started to pray while I was still in the office. After talking and praying with my mom, I felt such a peace and reassurance that everything was going to be okay. GOD IS SO AMAZING!!!

In order to gain new clients, I was in the process of meeting families. One day I went to meet a new client who had a baby, and she needed someone to watch him. After the meeting we talked on the phone to try to work out our schedules. After thinking over the conversation, I realized it just confirmed that I needed go back home, and I honestly believed it was so that my business could flourish. Job 23:10 (NIV) says, *"But he knows the way that I take; when he has tried me, I will come forth as gold."*

With everything going on, I was struggling mentally, physically, and spiritually. Then the holidays came, and Thanksgiving was good. My parents then came to visit for Christmas. During that visit, my parents were so concerned about my health that my dad was ready for me to come home with them that weekend. Earlier in the day we had taken a trip to the beach, and while walking on the beach, I had started throwing up. I told them that I had a dance conference in February, and I couldn't miss it. It was nothing but God's grace and mercy that got me through rehearsals and other ministry events over those next couple of months. I was also packing up my apartment and preparing to move during this time, which was hard. I was really blessed that my friend and her children helped me pack and clean my apartment.

February came, and I ministered at the conference with the rest of the dance ministry. I know it was only God that got me through that weekend. After that conference I went to my sister's house to finish packing up to move back to Pennsylvania. This was a very surreal moment because I never imagined myself moving back to Pennsylvania. I felt settled in North Carolina, and I had friends and had gotten closer to the family that was there.

Even though I was in a season where my body was not 100 percent, I knew God would keep His promise that no weapon formed against me would prosper, no sickness or disease come by my dwelling. The Bible says that God's Word *"will not return to me empty"* (NIV, Isaiah 55:11). This means that when God sends His word, it must accomplish the goal it was sent for.

The God we serve is a promise keeper. I finished packing, and my mother and I were on our way back to Pennsylvania.

Ezekiel 12: 28 (NIV) says, "*Therefore say to them, 'This is what the Sovereign Lord says: None of my words will be delayed any longer; whatever I say will be fulfilled, declares the Sovereign Lord.'*" And get this: the God we serve is so thorough that he even watches to see that his word is fulfilled, as stated in Jeremiah 1:12 (NIV).

CHAPTER 3

P.R.A.I.S.E. in the Fire

As I mentioned in the previous chapter, I wasn't 100%, but I was trusting and believing God's Word, I was already healed, whole, complete, but I just needed to walk in the victory God had already given me. You may also be in a season where you are waiting for the manifestation of your complete healing, be it mentally, physically, emotionally, etc., but don't know how to walk in the faith that God has already made you victorious. Here is what God gave me concerning walking in the victory that God has already given us: we must PRAISE, which is an acronym for Pray, Repent, Abstain, Intercession, Surrender, Elevate.

The first letter in the acronym is P, which stands for Pray. What is prayer? Prayer is simply a conversation with God. To walk in victory, we must be intentional about our prayer life. It is important to set aside time to spend with the Father in prayer without distractions. In Matthew 6:5-13, Jesus, in His sermon on the mount, gave the crowd instructions on prayer. His first instruction was not to be like the hypocrites who pray only to be seen but instead go into your room and close the door (get rid of distractions) and pray to the Father who is not seen. Jesus then says when the Father sees what you have done in secret, he will reward you.

Jesus's next instruction on how to pray was not to babble. Matthew 6:7-8 (NIV) says, *"And when you pray, do not keep on babbling like pagans, for they think they will be heard because of their many words. Do not be like them, for your Father knows what you need before you ask him."* So basically, Jesus is saying you don't have to use a lot of words when praying because God already knows what you need before you ask. So do not be intimidated by others you hear pray who use a lot of words.

In Matthew 6:9 Jesus tells us how we ought to pray and then recites the Lord's Prayer. The Lord's Prayer is not just a prayer but a blueprint/template for us to use to model our prayers. You can do this by using the acronym A.C.T.S.: Acknowledgement, Confession, Thanksgiving, Supplication. First, *A*cknowledge the Father and who He is when you come into his presence for, he is Holy, and he is King. *"Our Father in heaven, hallowed be your name."*

Confession is next. Not only should we ask God to forgive us, but we must also forgive others. *"And forgive us our debts, as we also have forgiven our debtors.*" We will be looking at repentance later, but we must realize that, to be truly victorious, we have to forgive.

Thanksgiving follows Confession. As we pray, not only should we pray with an attitude of thanksgiving but we should also thank God for everything He has done for us. In the Lord's Prayer the words do not outwardly tell the Father thank you, but Philippians 4:6 (NIV) says, "*Do not be anxious about anything, but in every situation, by prayer and petition, with thanksgiving, present your requests to God.*" 1 Thessalonians 5:18 (NIV) says, "*Do not be anxious about anything, but in every situation, by prayer and petition, with thanksgiving, present your requests to God.*

Supplication is the last word in the A.C.T.S. acronym. Supplication is simply asking God for what you want. Going back to the Lord's Prayer, we find several examples. One is the request that "*your kingdom come, your will be done, on earth as it is in heaven.*" Another example in the Lord's prayer is "*Give us today our daily bread.*" So whatever you need--healing, peace, joy, wisdom, provision, etc.--you can ask the Father.

The next letter in PRAISE is R, which stands for Repent. What does it mean to repent? Simply put, to repent means to sincerely regret and be remorseful for any wrongdoings and then to turn away from those things and return to God. It is not simply asking God for forgiveness. Repentance requires a shift not only in behavior but also in mind. God wants us to come to Him to repent, but in our repentance, we must do a 180-degree shift away from sin and not return to that sin but turn to God. Matthew 3:8 (Amplified Bible) says, *"So produce fruit that is consistent with repentance [demonstrating new behavior that proves a change of heart, and a conscious decision to turn away from sin]."*

In Ezekiel 18 the Lord speaks through the prophet Ezekiel to the Israelites about being righteous and how those who are righteous will live and those who sin will die. Verses 21 and 22 (NIV) say, *"But if a wicked person turns away from all the sins they have committed and keeps all my decrees and does what is just and right, that person will surely live; they will not die. None of the offenses they have committed will be remembered against them. Because of the righteous things they have done, they will live."* Verses 30-32 say, *"Therefore, you Israelites, I will judge each of you according to your own ways, declares the Sovereign Lord. Repent! Turn away from all your offenses; then sin will not be your downfall. Rid yourselves of all the offenses you have committed, and get a new heart and a new spirit. Why will you die, people of Israel? For I take no pleasure in the death of anyone, declares the Sovereign Lord. Repent and live!"*

In Luke 15:7 (NIV) Jesus says to the Pharisees and the teachers of the law, *"I tell you that in the same way there will be more rejoicing in heaven over one sinner who repents than over ninety-nine righteous persons who do not need to repent."* So Jesus would rather us repent as sinners than *think* we're righteous and not repent.

The A in PRAISE stands for Abstain. Merriam-Webster's definition of the word "abstain" is this: "to choose not to do or have something: to refrain deliberately and often with an effort of self-denial from an action or practice." It gives as an example "abstain from drinking." 1 Peter 2:11 (NIV) says, *"Dear friends, I urge you, as foreigners and exiles, to abstain from sinful desires, which wage war against your soul."* As believers in Jesus Christ, we should choose to stay away from those things that are contrary to the fruits of the spirit in order to walk in victory. Sometimes God will call us to abstain from certain things to bring us closer to Him. This may mean that we must abstain from things like food (fasting), alcohol/and or drugs, sex, social media, and television. 1 Thessalonians 5:22 (NIV) simply says to *"reject every kind of evil."* Am I telling you not to use Facebook or not to watch television? No, but if what you are doing is taking your focus away from God and causing you to spend less and less time with the Father, then it is probably a great idea to abstain from those things.

The next letter in PRAISE. is I, which stands for Intercession
. Merriam-Webster defines intercession as follows: the act of
interceding also: prayer, petition, or entreaty in favor of another.
Galatians 6:2 (NIV) tells us to *"carry each other's burdens,
and in this way you will fulfill the law of Christ."* When we
intercede, we are praying to God on behalf of others, and it
is important that we pray for one another. In 1 Timothy 2:1
(ESV) Paul says, *"First of all, then, I urge that supplications,
prayers, intercessions, and thanksgivings be made for all people."*
So not only should we be interceding for those close to us, but
we should also be interceding for those around us such as our
neighbors, our government officials, our teachers...anyone we
may encounter daily. James 5:16 (NIV) says, *"Therefore confess
your sins to each other and pray for each other so that you may be
healed. The prayer of a righteous person is powerful and effective."*
So just by standing in the gap for someone else, you may help
them receive the healing they need, the miracle they need, the
deliverance they need. And above all they may ask that God
comes into the heart and to become their Lord and Savior.

As the Bible urges us to intercede for others, it also lets us
know that we have the best two intercessors interceding for
us. The first one is Jesus Christ, who is our intercessor in
heaven. Hebrews 7:24-25 (NIV) says, *"But because Jesus lives
forever, he has a permanent priesthood. Therefore he is able to*

save completely those who come to God through him, because he always lives to intercede for them.".

Our second intercessor is the Holy Spirit, who is our intercessor on earth. Romans 8:26 (NIV) says, *"In the same way, the Spirit helps us in our weakness. We do not know what we ought to pray for, but the Spirit himself intercedes for us through wordless groans."* Intercession can help us walk in victory, because as we intercede for others, we are building our faith by believing that God will intervene in someone else's situation.

The next letter is S, which stands for Surrender. Merriam-Webster's definition of "surrender" is as follows: "to yield to the power, control, or possession of another upon compulsion or demand." If we truly want to live victoriously regardless of our situation, we must surrender completely to the Father. We must surrender to God's will and His way. Not worrying and casting your cares upon the Lord is you giving up control and allowing God to have His way. Even when we do not understand it, we must trust and have faith that God will do and provide what is best for us. 1 Peter 5:7 (NIV) says, *"Cast all your anxiety on him because he cares for you."* God cares about everything that concerns you, no matter how big or small. And Matthew 6:34 (NIV) reminds us not to worry: *"Therefore do not worry about tomorrow, for tomorrow will worry about itself. Each day has enough trouble of its own ."*

Proverbs 3:5-6 (NIV) encourages you to *"trust in the Lord with all your heart and lean not on your own understanding; in all your ways submit to him, and he will make your paths straight."* Even when we do not understand it, we must trust and have faith that God will do and provide what is best for us. In our humanity, it is hard to give up control, especially when we do not know the plan, and sometimes we pick and choose which parts of our life we will surrender. For example, you may surrender all your and anxieties and cares when it comes to your health but not when it comes to your finances or relationships. Jeremiah 29:11 (NIV) states, *"'For I know the plans I have for you,' declares the Lord, 'plans to prosper you and not to harm you, plans to give you hope and a future.'"* Saints, God wants all of us, so when you choose to surrender to the Father (which I pray you do), I urge you to surrender EVERYTHING because God already knows what you need.

The last letter in the PRAISE acronym is E, which stands for Elevate. Even though we are talking about being victorious, we must also remember that, because of Jesus Christ and His great sacrifice for us, the victory has already been won. Our goal is to walk in the victory that has already been given to us. Deuteronomy 20:4 (NIV) says, *"For the Lord your God is the one who goes with you to fight for you against your enemies to give you victory."* When I think of the word "elevate," I think of an eagle, so I did some research, and what I found was so amazing and revelatory. One way that eagles can gain altitude is, rather than using their wings and flapping, relying on rising air currents. But these aren't normal air currents. According to American Ornithological Society, thermal updrafts allow eagles to soar higher compared to orographic updrafts. Thermal updrafts are rising air currents that occur when energy from the sun heats air at the Earth's surface and causes it to rise. The eagle then uses this hot air to gain altitude (i.e., to ELEVATE) (Aos Fly like an eagle).

Just as the eagle uses the upward movement of the heated air to rise, sometimes God allows us to be amid the fire, and while we feel the heat as children of God, we must allow the pressure and heat of our circumstances to elevate our faith. We must ride on the upward current of our faith and the wind of the Holy Spirit and soar above any situation. Remember that the above source said INSTEAD of flapping the eagle relies on rising air currents (Aos Fly like an eagle). That statement is very powerful because it speaks to the fact that God has already given us the tools and paved the way and has already provided what we need to overcome any circumstance.

I can use my testimony to illustrate how God has provided everything we need to overcome. God had already given me a measure of faith; He had already put the right medical team in place and put the right people in my circle to pray with me and for me. All those things together certainly helped and continue to help me overcome. But even though God provided those things, my main reliance, dependency, and trust had to be on God Himself. Just like the eagles relied on the current, as children of God we must place our true reliance and dependency on the Father because we only overcome because Jesus overcame first. 1 John 5:4 (NIV) says, "*For everyone born of God overcomes the world. This is the victory that has overcome the world, even our faith.*"

One definition Merriam-Webster gives for "elevate" is "to improve morally, intellectually, or culturally." To walk in our victory, we must improve our prayer life and our level of repentance. We must improve our thinking about the things we listen to and watch and even the people we allow around us. If they are not bearing fruit and are causing us to sin, then we should avoid interacting with them . We should improve the way we intercede for others. We must improve our level of surrender to God, and when we do these things, God will ELEVATE us.

CHAPTER 4

Forged in the Fire

As I stated before, I moved back to my parents' house after the conference, which was an adjustment. My parents now had two (soon to be three) toddlers living in their home. I still wasn't sure why God had me return home. I just kept asking Him what He would have me do here. I truly thought that my coming home had something to do with getting my childcare business going, but at that moment I wasn't physically able to run a daycare. I came home in February 2020, and it took me a few weeks to adjust to living back at home with my parents and having two toddlers running around. I then started the process of finding physicians so that my health situations could be addressed. Because the previous cardiologist had thought I had a hole in my heart and because my blood pressure was not under control, the first doctor I needed to find was a cardiologist. This process was hard; I didn't even know where to begin, but God knew exactly who to put into place. I thought and prayed about where to find a cardiologist. One day I was just googling, and I came across a cardiology practice with great reviews, so I decided to call them. At this time we were starting to hear more and more about Covid-19. The number of cases was continuing to go up, so states were shutting down and limiting the number of people in buildings, including medical offices . Nevertheless, I made an appointment with the cardiologist in March. Little did I know the heat was about to be turned up. I called the day before my appointment just to make sure what the Covid protocols were before I brought someone with me. The administrator I spoke to told me that everything was fine and that they would see me the next day. My parents and I got to the appointment, and there was no one there except the front desk administrator and a couple of nurses.

The doctor I was supposed to see was a female. I got to the desk and gave the receptionist my information. She then asked me for the information a second time and said, "We might have skipped you; we've been calling patients to reschedule appointments due to Covid." So instead of sending me home, she called the head doctor of the practice, who was working down the street at the hospital. He came and looked at me. He looked through my test from North Carolina and said he wanted to run all new tests. He also added other tests on top of those. HALLELUJAH! He then said to me, "You're too young to be having these issues."

By the end of the month, I was in the hospital getting a heart catheterization. My blood pressure was so high that they kept me in the hospital. I was there for a week. While I was in the hospital, they did a lot of tests, some of which I had never heard of. God knew just what to do and who He wanted to use. Test after test failed to show a hole in my heart. Glory be to God. I was then put on the right combination of blood pressure medicine plus a diuretic. We finally found out that my kidneys were not working the way they should. My kidneys were working at only 15%, which explained the symptoms I was having.

So now that my blood pressure was pretty much under control, my cardiologist referred me to a nephrologist (a kidney doctor). I went to see him, and he went over my bloodwork. He said that my numbers were not where they were supposed to be. However, they were stable, which was a blessing! He also said we would watch and see if my numbers remained stable. My blood pressure was under control, but the medication I was on was a high dosage, and one of them would make me extremely sleepy. I would always take a nap after taking that medication, but I would still struggle to stay awake at work. I couldn't wait to get home so that I could go to sleep.

I had about three more visits with the kidney doctor, and the last visit he said, "Well, Ms. LaRue, I am going to refer you for a kidney transplant." My whole attitude changed. I wasn't expecting to hear that. I had never had a surgery before, and I was scared. I was confused and asked myself how I'd reached that point. I prayed and continued to ask God to help me, and I thanked Him every day. I even told God that I was scared and that I didn't know what to do. I hadn't told anyone other than my parents and my older sister at this point. The doctor then left me a number with a nurse coordinator's name, which was Bernadine. It took me about two weeks to I call her.

God tends to use our trials to build our faith. 1 Peter 1:6,7 (King James Version) tells us to rejoice *"that the trial of your faith, being much more precious than of gold that perisheth, though it be tried with fire, might be found unto praise and honour and glory at the appearing of Jesus Christ."* Even though I was going through a trial, I believed God was molding me and allowing me to feel that pressure because He wanted to make me come out as pure gold. I still had to remember to think about the positive things. Most of us have heard or read Philippians 4:4-9 (NIV), which reads *"Rejoice in the Lord always; again I will say, rejoice! Let your gentle spirit be known to all people. The Lord is near. Do not be anxious about anything, but in everything by prayer and pleading with thanksgiving let your requests be made known to God. And the peace of God, which surpasses all comprehension, will guard your hearts and minds in Christ Jesus. Finally, brothers and sisters, whatever is true, whatever is honorable, whatever is right, whatever is pure, whatever is lovely, whatever is commendable, if there is any excellence and if anything worthy of praise, think about these things. As for the things you have learned and received and heard and seen in me, practice these things, and the God of peace will be with you."*

I held on to scripture. Yes, I still had my moments. Some lasted longer than others, but through it all, I held on to Philippians 4:4-9 and thought about why I was still here; God must have a plan and a purpose for me. I kept thinking about how no one (including myself) knew how sick I was, how He protected me, kept me, and shielded me. And it was prayers from all my family, especially my mother and my close circle of friends. I encourage those who are going through experiences like this to remember and look back at God's goodness and mercy in their lives and think of those things that are right, pure, lovely, and praiseworthy.

It took me two weeks to call Bernadine. She then gave me a call back and explained that my kidney doctor wanted me to get a transplant because even though I was stable, they wanted to prevent things from worsening. And the fact that I was not on dialysis was a plus. I forgot to mention that even though the doctor said my kidneys were functioning at 15%, I was not on dialysis. You can't tell me God isn't good! While I was on the phone with Ms. Bernadine, I was emotional because we started to schedule my transplant evaluation so that I could get approved to get on the transplant list.

Ms. Bernadine went over my options regarding the choice between a living donor and a non-living donor. However, the transplant list was about five years long if you do not have a living donor. As she was going over everything, I began feeling more overwhelmed because it started to become real. As I was talking to Bernadine and feeling sad and overwhelmed, my mom happened to pull up to the house and saw me crying, and I just handed my mom the phone. She talked to Bernadine for a while and then handed me back the phone. I calmed down and was able to continue the conversation. Ms. Bernadine informed me that a pre-transplant coordinator would contact me to set up a pre-transplant evaluation. After the conversation, I talked to my parents and my mom prayed for me. My dad told me everything would be fine and that we just had to do what we had to do. It made me feel a little better knowing that my parents were being supportive.

CHAPTER 5

In the Middle of the Fire

After I spoke to Bernadine the next day, I decided to tell the rest of my siblings. This was super hard for me. I was still trying to process everything. I also didn't want to worry or upset my siblings. When I told them, they were supportive and asked what they could do and what the next steps were. I told them that I had to have a transplant evaluation to see whether I would be a good candidate for the transplant list.

The next step was my transplant evaluation. I was very happy, surprised, and thankful that two of my sisters, Tyesha and Zykia, traveled from their homes to be with me during my evaluation. The evaluation was an all-day event. I spoke to different members of the transplant team. I saw the pre-op transplant coordinator, transplant doctor, surgeon, nutritionist, and a finance person. I also had to get a couple of tests done while I was there. I had to get lab work and an ultrasound. Let me tell you--getting that lab work was a victory all on its own. I had to give 18 tubes of blood that day. That was a big deal for me because I don't do well with needles. God has truly helped me with my fear and anxiety, especially when it comes to needles and getting blood drawn. I still get a little nervous when new people draw my blood, but overall, my reaction is a lot better.

The transplant team went over what would happen once I was on the transplant list, what I would have to do to stay on the list, and the pre- and post-operative procedures. During the evaluation I was also given some ideas on how to reach out to people to see if anyone would be willing to donate. I was provided with a website where friends and family could register to be a potential donor.

In the days that followed my evaluation, I started reaching out to my siblings and family to provide them with the website address to register as a potential donor. I can honestly say that even though I was listening to the members of the transplant team, I was getting a little upset because this was getting to be more and more of a reality. I was still in disbelief that I was in this situation and was really in the process of getting put on the transplant list. I had seen people get transplants on medical shows and heard of people in need of a transplant of some sort and miraculously receive a donated organ, but I never thought that I would be in a situation where I needed one.

I had to get three more tests done before my case would be brought before the transplant committee, which would decide if I was eligible to be on the United Network for Organ Sharing (UNOS) list. I had to have an echocardiogram and a stress test and see my gynecologist. I scheduled and completed these tests and sent them to the transplant committee by the third week in November. (Remember we were still in Covid lockdown, so everything was a little slower.) The holidays were just around the corner. Thanksgiving was quiet and nice. I was still going to work and helping with the kids as much as I could.

In addition to feeling anxious about the transplant process, I was still working at the gym, and our gym was opening more and more to the public. I started to get anxious about the Covid precautions because I didn't want to take the risk of getting sick, especially since I was so close to finding a match and having my transplant surgery. But I relied on three certainties: God cannot lie, His word is true, and He takes care of His children. One of my favorite verses in scripture is Matthew 6:26 (NIV): *"Look at the birds of the air; they do not sow or reap or store away in barns, and yet your heavenly Father feeds them. Are you not much more valuable than they?"* This verse really helped me to remember that, even in this climate, God was still going to take care not only of me but also my family. If He takes care of the birds, you know how much more He take care of us.

And that's exactly what He did. He helped me with my job. I went to my boss and stated my concerns and asked her if I could be put on a shift where I didn't have to interact with as many people, and she put me on a shift that the flow of traffic was a lot less. God truly took care of me while I worked at the gym, and I didn't get sick--PRAISE GOD--even when I had coworkers get sick. I continued to work and started to prepare for what the next steps were in this process.

That season of waiting and preparation was very hard and often very lonely. Even though I had told family and friends, who were very supportive about going to doctor's appointments with me, registering to be a donor, etc., I still felt very lonely emotionally. It was hard because internally I was dealing with a lot of anxiety and was very scared. I felt like I couldn't talk to anyone (other than God) about what I was feeling on the inside. I just felt like no one had time or wanted to listen to everything that was going on inside me. The transplant team would send me stuff in the mail, and I just wanted to sit down with someone and go through the information I received. I felt this way because even though I had supportive family and friends, they really didn't understand all that was going on with me. Neither I nor my immediate family had ever dealt with anything like this. Like I mentioned before, I had never had a surgery before, so with this being my first surgery and a major one at that, I just felt like no one truly understood whenever I would get emotional. That wasn't anyone's fault because they had never been in this position, but it left me feeling lonely.

Another thing that made me anxious was the fact that Covid numbers were increasing and my family was having different celebrations which I chose not to attend just to be precautious. In those times when I would start to feel overwhelmed, anxious, and lonely, I would just go into my room and cry, but every time I would start to cry, I would hear the Holy Spirit whisper, "I'm with you." I would then wipe my face, and I would feel a peace. God's presence and the still small voice of the Holy Spirit gave me the encouragement and the push that I needed to keep going. And God's Word is so true. Not only through this journey but throughout my entire life, God has shown me time and time again that He is always with me and that, in spite of my feelings or the situation, I can always rely on Him. And let me tell you--while people in their humanity are very inconsistent and unreliable, the Lord God Almighty is very consistent, and He can't fail or lie.

God was also very gracious and loving in blessing me with an amazing group of prayer warriors and intercessors. I want to take time and emphasize the importance of having a relationship with God for yourself but also of having people around you in your circle that will pray, intercede, and stand in the gap for you, and boy oh boy did I have that! I can't thank God enough for the men and women who prayed for me. I truly love and appreciate them all. The word of God says we are to pray for one another. God truly answers prayers, and James 5:16 (The Message) says, *"Make this your common practice: Confess your sins to each other and pray for each other so that you can live together whole and healed."* The prayer of a person living right with God is something powerful to be reckoned with. An example of this is Job 42:10 (KJV): *"And the Lord turned the captivity of Job, when he prayed for his friends: also the Lord gave Job twice as much as he had before."*

Although it is very important that we pray for our close friends and family, it is just as important to pray for those we do not know in a personal way. God wants us to love others as we love ourselves, and part of loving somebody is being able to pray for them. Jesus said, *"Truly I tell you that if two of you on earth agree about anything they ask for, it will be done for them by my Father in heaven. For where two or three gather in my name, there am I with them"* (NIV, Matthew 18: 19-20). Surround yourself with prayer warriors and certainly be your own prayer warrior first and foremost. I also encourage you, as you are going through your own battles and circumstances, to make sure you take time to pray for others because you not only increase your faith but can also help strengthen someone else's faith, someone who may not have the strength or the words to say. I had moments where my faith was not strong, and I was able to call and talk to one of my prayer warriors. They would pray and encourage me, which really helped increase my faith. I know many of my family and friends put me on prayer lists at their churches, and I also joined a prayer group that meets every morning at 7 a.m. That prayer group was a tremendous blessing to me, and my mom even started to join in. Prayer helped get me through one of the most difficult times of my life

December 2020 came, and the Wednesday before Christmas I was just sitting on my couch watching TV when I received a phone call that I was approved and on the transplant list. I was so excited that after I hung up the phone, I screamed with happiness. I couldn't and still can't thank God enough for his faithfulness towards me. I couldn't wait to tell my family about the great news. After I told my family, all I could think was that one more step was completed and I needed to know the next step. The lady I spoke with on that phone call asked me if I had any living donors, and I did have family members who said they would register to be donors. I didn't have the ability to see who had done it. I only knew of those who personally told me they had.

I was so excited. I felt like we had gotten through a big part of this process, but the process was not nearly over. Once I settled down, I asked God, "What is the next step, Lord?" and "Who is going to be my donor?" I had never had surgery before, and this was going to be a big one. The next question was what surgery was going to be like. In the days that followed, I talked to some more family members and also sent the registration information to other family members and friends.

A few weeks later, my sister called and said she had an appointment for her evaluation scheduled for the first week in February. That was amazing, and I was super excited because that meant someone who registered was contacted and that the next portion of the transplant process could start. I am so very thankful for my sister, and this was amazing because no one else had informed me that they were scheduled for an evaluation.

Near the end of February, I received a call. I thought it was my coordinator telling me my sister was approved, but it was my social worker. Curious, I called my sister and asked her if she had heard anything, and she said no. I told her she should probably call and find out what was going on. She then called and then called me back and said she'd been approved. I screamed and cried and just thanked God because He continued to show faithfulness to me. We then scheduled the transplant surgery for April 2 (which I didn't find out until later was Good Friday).

For the subsequent weeks, I got bloodwork done once a week and was still working. Around this time, I started noticing something happening to my skin. It became very itchy and started peeling. It also became very dry and extremely tight and painful. I also dark spots on my body, mainly on my legs and arms. My skin became so itchy. One night it was so unbearable and I was so scared that I couldn't sleep. I actually went and woke my mom up crying. At first she looked at my skin, and then she started to pray, and the Holy Spirit led her to tell me to get a specific soap. After we prayed, I was able to go to sleep. The next day I went and got the soap. After a couple of weeks, I was able to notice a big difference in my skin.

The end of March came, and before I knew it, it was the day before surgery. My brother, sister, and my sister's fiancé (now her husband) came to Pennsylvania to be with us. We all had a great time just hanging out, talking in the hotel room, and playing cards. As the night progressed, I started to get a little anxious. I had never had surgery before, but I was excited about being able to feel better after the surgery, even though I was nervous about all the needles and tubes that come with being in the hospital.

I finally fell asleep. We got up around 5:00 am because we had to be at the hospital by 6:00 am. When we got there, they called my sister Zykia first. They then called me back. We were both in the same holding area. She was right across from me. I remember I just kept telling her I loved her and asking her if she was okay.

I knew she was doing this out of love, and I didn't want her in any more pain than necessary. My sister was a soldier that day. She was very tough through it all. Then after the nurse asked us questions, we got into our gowns, and they inserted my IV. The nurses then rolled my sister to the holding area where they would start giving us our pre-surgery anesthesia. One of the nurses then rolled me down, and my sister and I were side by side. I was nervous, but I knew God had everything under control.

They rolled my sister off to begin her surgery and later took me to mine. At that point I wasn't aware of what was going on. I started to fall asleep because of the anesthesia. By the time we hit the elevator, I was asleep. I woke up in recovery, and I was in a little pain. My family was able to come and see me, one person at a time. The recovery process had officially begun.

I found out that my sister was down the hall and around the corner from my room, which was amazing. About three days after surgery, the doctors and nurses started getting me up and moving and walking the hallway. I believe my sister was discharged that same day, and I was able to walk down to her room and sit with her and my brother in-law before she went back home.

I stayed in the hospital for three more days because I had two drain bulbs and the doctors wanted to make sure the amount of fluid that was draining had significantly decreased and that

that I could use the bathroom without issue before leaving. As I mentioned previously, prior to surgery I was having issues with my skin. But the nurses were now complimenting me on how soft my skin was. I was finally discharged from the hospital, but instead of going home, we stayed at a lodging facility for patients and their families who travel to the area and are receiving medical care. I would have to see the doctor every couple of days after surgery, and I lived one and a half hours away.

After getting settled in, I was very sore, although that first night my pain level wasn't bad. My mom and I still prayed for me and for those in the rooms around us. My mom would walk with me up and down the hallway so that I could build some strength. I then had my post-op visit two days after discharge, and my bloodwork numbers were low. I was a little concerned about that, but the doctors weren't particularly concerned and told me my numbers would increase and level over time. In the meantime, I continued to pray and believe God for complete healing.

The next post-op appointment was a couple of days later, and some of my numbers increased a little, but the doctors started talking to me about possibly having to have a blood transfusion. They wanted to wait for one more visit to make that decision. The evening before my next appointment, I remember not feeling the greatest. The following morning, the morning of my appointment, I did feel a little weak, but I kept pushing through. I got to meet my first post-op coordinator after having my blood drawn. As she was talking to my mom and me, another lady came in and handed her a sticky note. She then told us that my red blood cell count was very low and that they were taking me down the hall to another section of the hospital. My coordinator asked me if I had fallen or cut myself, and I told her no.

The nurses rushed me to a room and started to prep me for the blood transfusion by starting the IV line (which even though my anxiety and nervousness with blood draws was better getting an IV was a different story) I screamed and cried because it was painful, and I was still processing the fact that I was about to get a blood transfusion, something that I have never had to experience before this. While I was crying, I remember asking my mom, "Why is this happening to me?" I also remember repeatedly saying, "I don't understand!"

But even during all that, I heard the Holy Spirit say, "I am with you," and I started to calm down and breathe. I was even able to call my older sister back and have a whole conversation. The God I serve is so amazing, and the mere fact that I was on God's mind in that moment gave me such a peace. Psalm 8:4 (NIV) says, *"What is mankind that you are mindful of them, human beings that you care for them?"* God was taking care of me in the middle of my anxiety, in the middle of the physical pain of the IV, and in the middle of all the questions that I had. And if you are reading this, I want to take a moment to let you know that GOD IS WITH YOU. He is Emmanuel (God with us), so you can trust and have faith that no matter what the situation, be it physical, emotional, or mental, you can call on Emmanuel, and He is there.

After the IV was hooked up, we had to wait for the blood to be transported over. The doctor said they were going to give me one unit of blood to see how I tolerated that and then would determine whether they would give me the second unit that day or another day. Once again God was right there fighting all my battles because I received both units of blood in the same day with no side effects or issues. God kept and continues to keep His word.

When my mom and I went back to our room, I was feeling a lot better than I had been. The next day I started to have some severe and intense gastrointestinal issues and had a hard time using the bathroom, so we let the doctor know and were told to get some MiraLAX. We did that, and we prayed after I took some MiraLAX. I also drank some hot lemon water, and within three days the pain completely went away. Thank you, Lord!!

After a few more visits, my doctors said it was okay for me to go home. As my mom and I were riding the shuttle back to our room, a Caucasian woman told us about her husband and how she had been there for months with him and that he needed a liver transplant and had some other medical issues. She talked about how she trusted God to heal her husband. Before we got off the shuttle, I prayed with her for her husband's healing and agreed with her that her husband would be healed. The next day my mom and I packed up our stuff and headed back home.

Going home was a relief, but I was a little nervous because, , This process completely new to me and my family s I had to do everything differently now, such as food preparation, and I had to pay extra close attention to the cleanliness of my environment. I was also and still am cautious about what I eat and drink.

Everything was going well. Two weeks after I had to go to my first post-op clinic visit, my doctors were truly impressed with the progress that I had made. I still had to get bloodwork twice a week. God is so very good because I was able to walk in and get my blood drawn without feeling overwhelming anxiety. God was still working on me when it came to not being anxious while waiting for the results.

I was healing very well and getting stronger every day. But an hour or two after returning from my next clinic visit, I went to the bathroom and found that one of my drain bulbs had fallen out. I yelled for my mom, who was upstairs, and then I yelled for my dad. I was so scared because I had a small open hole in my side where the tube was. My mom ran downstairs to see what had happened. At that moment, fear wanted to take over, but then my mom started praying. I called the clinic and told the nurse what had happened, and she asked if a lot of fluid was coming out of the site. I told her no. She then asked if we had some gauze, which we did. The nurse then said just to cover the site and keep it dry and that it would close on its own.

Within a week the hole had mostly closed. God is so good because He kept and protected me from infection, even though I was very scared. God never left me, and I told the Lord, "Lord, I know you didn't bring me this far to leave me." My mindset then changed from one of fear and anxiety to one centered on the thought, "God, I'm glad that the tube is gone because I can sleep more comfortably and I don't have to pour the bulb out multiple times." God is so amazing, and He truly cares about EVERYTHING that concerns us.

I continued to heal and to go to my appointments. I started to walk more and more, and there were times when I would start to get emotional while I was walking because months prior it was exhausting and hard for me to walk even short distances. I was now walking without being super exhausted, and although I did have some muscle soreness, I was just so grateful that I was moving and walking without feeling sick.

In July at my three-month visit, the doctors performed a biopsy. I really didn't know what to expect, but God's peace was with me. I was nervous, but my anxiety was very low, and any anxiety I did have was over getting the results rather than the actual procedure. The doctor came in later in the day to tell my mom and me the results, and he said my kidney numbers were better than his! No one can convince me that my God is not a healer or that He won't do *"exceeding abundantly above all that we ask or think, according to the power that worketh in us"* (KJV, Ephesians 3:20). God had really answered my prayers exceedingly and abundantly. As the next few months passed, I began to start moving around more. I was consistently walking, mowing the grass, running, and playing with my nieces and nephews, which was an absolute joy.

Luke 10:19 (AMP) says, *"Listen carefully: I have given you authority [that you now possess] to tread on [a]serpents and scorpions, and [the ability to exercise authority] over all the power of the enemy (Satan); and nothing will [in any way] harm you."* And I would find out just how true this scripture is in December of 2021. The week between Christmas and New Year's Day, I started feeling unwell. I had a fever and just felt off. After talking to my parents, I went to the ER. After an initial evaluation, everything seemed okay, but I was having extreme back pain, so right before I was about to get released, the physician decided to have me tested for Covid. The test came back positive.

I started to get very upset at first because I believed I was being careful, and I had been vaccinated. I called a couple of my prayer warriors, and we prayed. Also, my transplant team stayed in contact with the ER staff the entire time, which was a blessing. My transplant team told me to stay very well hydrated and to isolate and to monitor my symptoms and breathing and to let them know if my symptoms got worse. I was also scheduled to have a monoclonal antibody infusion two days later. After receiving the infusion, I started to feel better. I was coughing some, but overall, I didn't feel bad. I had to isolate for three weeks, but I fully recovered! HALLELUJAH, I had overcome, and God had won another battle on my behalf. Many people with underlying conditions or health issues were passing away, but God's grace and mercy kept me.

CHAPTER 6

I Don't Smell Like Smoke

Battle after battle and struggle after struggle God has always been and will always be the fourth man in the fire fighting for me and protecting me. After all that I have gone through, I can truly say that I don't smell like smoke. As a matter of fact, I have gone from four blood pressure medications with high dosages three times a day to two low dosage medications, one twice a day and one once a day. I am also off a few other medications I was on. I had my one-year post- transplant biopsy, and everything looks very good. My sister is also doing well. Although parts of this journey were physically and emotionally painful, I believe that I needed to share my testimony so that it might boost the faith of others.

Right now I am almost two years post-transplant. Things are going very well. I still have moments of anxiety. But even during that, I remind myself that God hasn't given me a spirit of fear and that He didn't bring me this far just to stop, and then those moments don't last as long as they used to. God keeps His promises, and every word He speaks to me He will fulfill. God's Word says, "*When anxiety was great within me, your consolation brought me joy*" (NIV, Psalm 94:19). I would often imagine God hugging me, and I could hear the Spirit say, "It's going to be okay." I encourage you to let the Holy Spirit console you. Today, let Daddy God shower you with His love. When you allow God to love you and you hand over all your fears, worries, and anxious thoughts, He will turn every situation around for your good.

Even if you are struggling or have struggled with mental health issues or negative beliefs or thoughts about yourself, do not believe the lie that God cannot use you for His glory. If God made you, He also has a plan and a purpose that must be accomplished through you. David declares in Psalm 139:14 (NIV) that "*I praise you because I am fearfully and wonderfully made; your works are wonderful, I know that full well.*" Satan is a liar, and the Bible says he is the father of lies, and he puts those lies and negative thoughts in our heads. To combat those lies of the enemy and to keep from having negative thoughts, we have to consistently remind ourselves of what God says about us.

We ought to get the attitude like David that we will praise the Lord because we are fearfully and wonderfully made and that no negative words spoken to us, about us, or over us can change that. This is because we are sculpted by the Creator and God said of everything He made, "It is good." God is an amazing Father, better than any earthly parent. As our heavenly Father, He doesn't want to see His children hurting. Isaiah 66:13 (NIV) says, "*As a mother comforts her child, so will I comfort you....*" God is loving and gentle, so just continue to put your complete trust in Him because the moment we don't feel or hear God is the moment He's doing His best work in our lives.

The situations and circumstances that we go through can feel very heavy to us, and sometimes we feel like it is too much for us mentally, physically, and spiritually. Jesus tells us in Matthew 11:28-30 (NIV), "*Come to me, all you who are weary and burdened, and I will give you rest. Take my yoke upon you and learn from me, for I am gentle and humble in heart, and you will find rest for your souls. For my yoke is easy and my burden is light.*" Just give it to God, and He'll make everything all right.

Whenever we give our problems, cares, worries, and anxieties to God, we have to totally surrender to God, because God wants to heal us everywhere we hurt. Another lesson I learned through this journey is that sometimes those around us don't truly understand the pain we are in until something bad happens, but God is with us through it all, and He is the only one who truly understands because He created us! We also may have to remind ourselves that God doesn't need us to do

His wonderful works; he is GOD all by himself. But He loves us so much that Hebrews 12:1 (English Standard Version) says, "*Therefore, since we are surrounded by so great a cloud of witnesses, let us also lay aside every weight, and sin which clings so closely, and let us run with endurance the race that is set before us.*" I encourage whoever is reading this to surround yourself with believers in Christ who will pray and stand in the gap with you and for you. I thank God for the circle of people He placed in my life who prayed and lifted me and my situations up to God, because those prayers helped get me through some rough days. Also, being surrounded by like-minded believers will help you become strong in the Lord. It will help encourage you and build your faith. Hearing testimonies of God's goodness and faithfulness can stir up the atmosphere, and that stirring can help you build your faith. When we build our faith, that weight that we spoke about earlier begins to get lighter and lighter until there is nothing.

God's desire is for us to rest in Him, and when we give our cares to God, He will give us His *shalom*. He promised to keep us in perfect peace, as he said in Isaiah 26:3, if we keep our mind stayed on Him and continue to believe His word. Since our God overcame the world, we have also overcome. God wants to see His children victorious and has already given us the victory in every circumstance, but to walk in that victory is a whole other level. To walk in victory, we must PRAISE (Pray, Repent, Abstain, Intercede, Surrender, and Elevate).

In conclusion, I can honestly say that I don't look like what I've been through. GOD is faithful and wants to heal you, and He wants you to be whole. God is more than amazing, so read God's Word and remind God of His promises daily. If God can do it for me, I believe He can do it for anyone! From this moment on, don't allow the enemy to plant negative thoughts about you or your situation in your mind but tell yourself daily, "I WIN" and "LET'S RUN THIS RACE!" Because we have already WON! We just have to walk in it.

Grace and Peace

Works Cited

1. Duerr, Adam. "Fly Like an Eagle." American Ornithological Society, 9 Apr. 2019, americanornithology.org/fly-like-an-eagle/. Accessed 6 Sept. 2023.

2. "Every." Merriam-Webster.com Dictionary, Merriam-Webster, https://www.merriam-webster.com/dictionary/every. Accessed 6 Sep. 2023.

3. "Win." Merriam-Webster.com Dictionary, Merriam-Webster, https://www.merriam-webster.com/dictionary/win. Accessed 6 Sep. 2023.

4. "Abstain." Merriam-Webster.com Dictionary, Merriam-Webster, https://www.merriam-webster.com/dictionary/abstain. Accessed 6 Sep. 2023.

5. "Intercession." Merriam-Webster.com Dictionary, Merriam-Webster, https://www.merriam-webster.com/dictionary/intercession. Accessed 6 Sep. 2023.

6. "Surrender." Merriam-Webster.com Dictionary, Merriam-Webster, https://www.merriam-webster.com/dictionary/surrender. Accessed 6 Sep. 2023.

7. "Elevate." Merriam-Webster.com Dictionary, Merriam-Webster, https://www.merriam-webster.com/dictionary/elevate. Accessed 6 Sep. 2023.

www.ingramcontent.com/pod-product-compliance
Lightning Source LLC
Chambersburg PA
CBHW070942280326
41934CB00009B/1989